CW00499936

Keto Cookbook for Beginners

The complete beginner's guide 50 easy, delicious recipes to get you started with balanced eating plans.

2

Sommario

INTRODUCTION

The ketogenic diet focuses on all health and supports all aspects, not just weight loss. This book gives you the latest research to help you feel more empowered to make the changes that are right for you.

These recipes are great for keeping your body healthy and keeping the insulin in your body at an optimal level. Preventing diabetes, is critical to healthy living.

The central principle of the ketogenic diet is to maintain ketosis, a metabolic state that causes your body to burn fat for daily fuel instead of glucose derived from carbohydrates.

So let's not waste time and get in shape right away with these delicious recipes designed especially for newcomers, being easy and quick to prepare.

Are you ready to delight your palate?

Let's start.

CHAPTER ONE

Avocado Cloud Toast

Preparation Time: 11 Min | Cooking Time: 33 Min | Servings: 2

Ingredients

- ¼ teaspoon garlic powder
- 2 large eggs, separated
- Pinch cream of tartar
- ½ cup mayonnaise
- 1 ounce cream cheese, cubed
- 2 teaspoons fresh lemon juice
- Fresh cracked pepper, to taste
- 4 slices fresh tomato
- 1 large avocado
- Salt, to taste

Directions

1. Warm the oven to 300 degrees and line a baking sheet with parchment paper.

2. In a portable bowl, beat egg whites and cream of tartar with a hand mixer on medium speed until stiff peaks form, about 30 seconds.
3. In another bowl, whisk together cream cheese, egg yolk, and garlic powder until light-colored and well combined.
4. Fold the egg whites tenderly into the cream cheese mixture.
5. Pour the mixture into the pan in 4-inch circles, 1 to 2 inches apart.
6. Bake for 20 - 30 minutes until lightly browned. Keep an eye on the sandwiches while cooking. Then take it out from the oven and let it cool completely.
7. In a portable bowl, combine the mayonnaise and fresh lemon juice.
8. Open and pit the avocado, then cut it into quarters and slice thinly.
9. Grill the sandwiches and spread them with the mayonnaise mixture.
10. Garnish each sandwich with 1 tomato slice and 1 sliced avocado wedge.
11. Season with salt and pepper before serving

Nutritional Facts:

Calories: 665, Fat 66g, Cholesterol 225 mg, Carbohydrates 5g, Protein 10g

Bacon Cheddar Chive Omelet

Prep Time: 11 Min | Cooking Time: 35 Min | Servings: 2

Ingredients

- 2 large Eggs
- 2 slices Bacon, already cooked
- 2 stalks Chives
- Salt and Pepper, to taste
- 1 tsp. Bacon Fat
- 1 oz. Cheddar Cheese

Directions

1. Prepare all the ingredients and heat the pan over medium-low heat with the bacon fat. Add the eggs and season with chives, salt and pepper.
2. As soon as the edges start to solidify, add the bacon in the center and cook for 20-30 seconds and remove from the heat.
3. Top with cheese and fold the edges like a burrito. Turn and heat on the other side.
4. Serve immediately and enjoy!

Nutritional Facts:

Calories: 462, Fat 40g, Carbohydrates 1g, Protein 23g

Breakfast Taco with Cheesy Shells

Prep Time: 11 Min | Cooking Time: 15 Min | Servings: 2

Ingredients

- ½ cup shredded cheddar cheese
- 1 cup shredded mozzarella cheese
- 4 slices bacon
- 2 tablespoons heavy cream
- 6 large eggs
- Salt, to taste
- 1 small tomato, chopped
- ½ medium avocado, diced
- Pepper, to taste

Directions

1. Place a wooden spoon in a bowl and set it aside.
2. Heat a large skillet over medium-high heat.
3. In a portable bowl, combine the mozzarella and cheddar cheese.
4. Sprinkle ¼ cup of the cheese mixture in a circle in the center of the pan.
5. Let the cheese melt and brown; then turn and cook until the bottom is golden.
6. Utilize a spatula to remove the cheese from the pan and cover with a wooden spoon to cool in a taco shell; repeat for the rest of the cheese.

7. Cook the bacon in the same dish until crisp; then drain them on absorbent paper and chop them.
8. Grease another pan and heat over medium-high heat.
9. In a handy bowl, whisk together the eggs, cream, salt and pepper.
10.　　Spout the eggs into the pan and cook for 3 to 5 minutes, stirring occasionally to stir.
11.　　Place the taco shells upright on two plates.
12.　　Pour the eggs into the shell; top with avocado, tomato and chopped bacon for serving.

Nutritional Facts:

Calories: 706, Fat 54g, Cholesterol 670 mg, Carbohydrates 9g, Protein 46g

Chocolate Chip Waffles

Prep Time: 15 Min | Cooking Time: 12 Min | Servings: 2

Ingredients

- 3 tablespoons low-carb vanilla protein powder
- 2 large eggs, separated
- 2 tablespoons unsalted butter, melted
- ½ teaspoon vanilla extract
- 1 tablespoon powdered erythritol
- Pinch salt
- Sugar-free maple syrup, to taste
- 2 tablespoons stevia-sweetened chocolate chips

Directions

1. In a portable bowl, beat the egg whites until stiff peaks form.
2. In another bowl, combine the protein powder, butter, egg yolks, erythritol, vanilla extract, and salt.
3. Add the egg whites to the protein powder mixture, then add the chocolate chips.
4. Grease and preheat a waffle iron, then cook the dough according to the manufacturer's instructions until golden brown.
5. Spot the waffles on a plate and garnish them with unsweetened maple syrup for serving.

Nutritional Facts:

Calories: 244, Fat 54g, Cholesterol 221 mg, Carbohydrates 3g, Protein 15g

Cinnamon Oatmeal

Prep Time: 13 Min | Cooking Time: 25 Min | Servings: 4

Ingredients

- 1 cup Crushed Pecans
- 3 1/2 cups Coconut Milk
- 3 oz. Cream Cheese
- 1/3 cup Flax Seed
- 1/2 cup Cauliflower, riced
- 1/3 cup Chia Seed
- 3 tbsp. Butter
- 1/4 cup Heavy Cream
- 3 tbsp. Erythritol powder
- 1/2 tbsp. Maple Flavor
- 1/2 tbsp. Cinnamon
- 10-15 drops Liquid Stevia
- 1/2 tsp. Vanilla
- 1/4 tsp. Nutmeg
- 1/4 tsp. All spice

Directions

1. Prepare the rice cauliflower in a food processor and set it aside. Heat the coconut milk in a pan over medium heat. Squash the nuts and add them to the pan over low heat until toasted.
2. Add the cauliflower to the coconut milk and bring to a boil. Reduce to a simmer and add the

spices and stir until combined. Add the erythritol powder to the pot. Add the stevia, flax and chia seeds.

3. Finally, add the butter, cream and cream cheese to the pan and mix again.
4. Serve immediately and enjoy!

Nutritional Facts:

Calories: 359, Fat 30.4g, Carbohydrates 5g, Protein 9.4g

Goat Cheese Frittata

Prep Time: 13 Min | Cooking Time: 30 Min | Servings: 4

Ingredients

- 2 tablespoons olive oil
- 16 medium spears asparagus
- 4 ounces sliced white mushrooms
- ½ cup heavy cream
- 12 large eggs
- 2 cloves minced garlic
- 2 green onions, sliced thin
- Pepper, to taste
- Salt, to taste
- 4 ounces crumbled goat cheese

Directions

1. Cut the ends of the asparagus and cut them into 2 inch pieces.
2. In a 10-inch cast-iron skillet, heat oil over medium-high heat.
3. Add the mushrooms and asparagus and sauté for 3-4 minutes until golden brown.
4. In a medium bowl, combine the eggs, cream, garlic, salt, and pepper.
5. Spout the liquid mixture into the pan and sprinkle with goat cheese and green onion.
6. Bake for 30 minutes at 375 degrees, until solid, then cut into quarters to serve.

Nutritional Facts:

Calories: 505, Fat 41g, Cholesterol 622 mg,
Carbohydrates 5g, Protein 28g

Jalapeno Cheddar Waffles

Prep Time: 25 Min | Cooking Time: 25 Min | Servings: 3

Ingredients

- 1 small Jalapeno
- 3 large Eggs
- 3 oz. Cream Cheese
- 1 tbsp. Coconut Flour
- 1 oz. Cheddar Cheese
- 1 tsp. Psyllium Husk Powder
- Salt and Pepper, to taste
- 1 tsp. Baking Powder

Directions

1. Combine all the ingredients with a blender until the mixture is smooth.
2. Prepare the waffle iron, and then pour in the waffle mix. Garnish with your favorite toppings.
3. Serve immediately and enjoy!

Nutritional Facts:

Calories: 337, Fat 27g, Carbohydrates 3g, Protein 16g

CHAPTER TWO

Apple Pecan Salad With Chicken

Prep Time: 11 Min | Cooking Time: 10 Min | Servings: 4

Ingredients:

- 2 chicken breasts
- 2 tablespoons vegetable oil
- 2 cups Romaine lettuce
- ¼ cup strawberries (sliced)
- 1 cup spinach
- ¼ cup cranberries (dried)
- ½ cup bleu cheese crumbles
- 2 tablespoons pecans (chopped)
- ¼ teaspoon black pepper
- ¼ teaspoon parsley (dried)
- ¼ teaspoon Himalayan sea salt
- ¼ teaspoon garlic powder

Directions:

1. Place a portable-sized pan on the stove and set the heat to medium-high. Add the oil to the pan and let it heat up.
2. While the pan is heating, take a small bowl and add the garlic powder, parsley, sea salt and black pepper. Stir until you get a homogeneous mixture.
3. Take each of the chicken breasts and sprinkle the powdered garlic mixture on all sides.
4. Place the seasoned chicken breast in the pan. Cook the chicken for five minutes, then turn it over and cook for another five minutes. Once the chicken's core temperature has reached 165 degrees Fahrenheit, remove it from the pan and let it sit on a cutting board.
5. While the chicken is resting, make the rest of the salad ready. In a large salad bowl, add the spinach, lettuce, strawberries and blueberries. Mix everything with the salad spoons. Divide the salad into two equal portions and top each portion with half the nuts and blue cheese.
6. Slice the chicken breast and put it on the salad. Serve with your favorite vinaigrette.

Nutritional Facts:

Calories 53, Carbs 5g, Fat 46g, Protein 24g

Avocado Tuna Melt Bites

Prep Time: 13 Min | Cooking Time: 3 Min | Servings: 2

Ingredients

- 1 medium Avocado, cubed
- 1 (10 oz.) Can Tuna, drained
- 1/2 cup Coconut Oil, for frying
- 1/4 cup Parmesan Cheese
- 1/3 cup Almond Flour
- 1/4 cup Mayonnaise
- Salt and Pepper, to Taste
- 1/2 tsp. Onion Powder
- 1/2 tsp. Garlic Powder

Directions

1. Add all ingredients except avocado and coconut oil to a bowl and mix.
2. Cut the avocado into cubes and mix it with the tuna. Form tuna balls and cover with almond flour.
3. Over medium Warm, heat the coconut oil in a pan. Once hot, add the tuna balls and sauté until golden brown.
4. Serve immediately and enjoy!

Nutritional Facts:

Calories: 135, Fat 11.8g, Carbohydrates 0.8g, Protein 6.2g

Buffalo Wild Wings Spicy Garlic Sauce Chicken Wings

Prep Time: 13 Min | Cooking Time: 50 Min | Servings: 4

Ingredients:

- ½ teaspoon Himalayan sea salt
- 2 ½ pounds chicken wings

For Sauce:

- ½ cup hot sauce
- ¼ cup avocado oil
- 2 tablespoons garlic powder
- ½ teaspoon Stevia (liquid)
- ¼ teaspoon cayenne pepper

Directions:

1. Preheat the oven to 400 degrees Fahrenheit.
2. Dry the wings with a paper towel while the oven is preheating and place them on a wire rack. Dredge with sea salt and bake for 45 minutes.

3. After 45 minutes, turn the oven on to the grill and leave the wings in the oven for another 5 minutes to get them crispy.
4. While the wings cook, prepare the sauce. Combine avocado oil, hot sauce, garlic powder, cayenne pepper and liquid stevia in a blender. Mix until smooth, then transfer to a large bowl (the bowl should be large enough to accommodate all of the wings).
5. The moment you take the wings are out of the oven, transfer them to the bowl with the sauce. Discard the wings so that they are all well covered.

Nutritional Facts:

Calories 498, Carbs 4g, Protein 30g, Fat 39g

Cashew Chicken Stir-Fry

Prep Time: 13 Min | Cooking Time: 20 Min | Servings: 4

Ingredients

- 2 7-ounce bags Noodle Rice
- 1 teaspoon coconut oil
- Salt and pepper, to taste
- 1 pound boneless chicken thighs, chopped
- 2 tablespoons soy sauce
- 2 tablespoons canned coconut milk
- 2 cloves minced garlic
- 20 small spears asparagus, sliced
- 1 teaspoon chili garlic sauce, optional
- ½ cup whole cashews

Directions

1. Pour the noodle rice into a colander and rinse well with cold water.
2. Grease an enormous skillet with cooking spray and heat over medium heat.
3. Add the noodle rice and season with salt and pepper. Fry until hot.
4. In another pan, heat the coconut oil over medium heat.

5. Add the chicken to the coconut oil and cook until golden brown, stirring frequently about 4 to 5 minutes.
6. Pour the coconut milk and soy sauce into the pan with the chicken.
7. Add the asparagus, cashews, hot sauce and garlic and simmer for 6 to 8 minutes, stirring occasionally.
8. Add the noodle rice and simmer for 2 minutes until heated through.

Nutritional Facts:

Calories: 313, Fat 20g, Carbohydrates 11g, Protein 22g, Cholesterol 106 mg

Cheese Stuffed Bacon Hot Dogs

Prep Time: 10 Min | Cooking Time: 21 Min | Servings: 6

Ingredients

- 6 Hot Dogs
- 12 slices of Bacon
- Salt and Pepper, to Taste
- 2 oz. Cheddar Cheese
- 1/2 tsp. Garlic Powder
- 1/2 tsp. Onion Powder

Directions

1. Preheat the oven to 400 F.
2. Make a slit in each hot dog and insert the sliced cheese into the slits. Swath each hot dog in 2 slices of bacon each, and then secure the bacon with a toothpick.
3. Spot the hot dogs on a baking sheet, and then season the hot dogs. Bake for at least 35 to 40 minutes until golden brown. Serve immediately and enjoy your food!

Nutritional Facts:

Calories: 380, Fat 34.5, Carbohydrates 0.3g, Protein 17g

Cheeseburger Crepes

Prep Time: 11 Min | Cooking Time: 20 Min | Servings: 2

Ingredients

- 6 ounces 80 percent lean ground beef
- 2 tablespoons olive oil
- ½ small yellow onion, diced
- 1 tablespoon sugar-free ketchup
- 2 ounces cream cheese, softened
- 1 ounce shredded cheddar cheese
- 2 tablespoons mayonnaise
- 2 large eggs

Directions

1. On medium heat, cook the minced meat and onion for 5 minutes in a greased pan.
2. Stir in cheddar cheese, ketchup and mayonnaise; then pour into a bowl and set aside.
3. In a medium bowl, make a paste by beating the eggs and cream cheese until smooth and well combined.
4. Grease an enormous skillet and heat over high heat.
5. Pour about half of the batter into the pan, tilt it to coat evenly and cook for 2 minutes.

6. Gently flip the pancake and fry for another 2 minutes, until lightly browned.
7. Remove the pancake on a plate and keep warm while you use the rest of the batter.
8. Pour cheeseburger mixture into pancakes and roll up; then cut in half to serve.

Nutritional Facts:

Calories: 600, Fat 53g, Carbohydrates 7g, Protein 27g, Cholesterol 291 mg

Chicken Lettuce Wraps

Prep Time: 13 Min | Cooking Time: 20 Min | Servings: 3

Ingredients:

- 1 pound chicken (ground)
- 1 tablespoon avocado oil
- 1 head of butter lettuce
- 3 green onions (sliced)
- 2 cups shiitake mushrooms (chopped)
- ¼ teaspoon black pepper
- ½ cup jicama (diced)
- ¼ teaspoon Himalayan sea salt
- 2 teaspoons onion powder

For Sauce:

- 2 cloves of garlic (minced)
- 1 tablespoon sesame oil
- ½ teaspoon ginger (grated)
- 1 tablespoon almond butter
- 3 tablespoons coconut aminos
- ½ tablespoon erythritol (sweetener)
- 1 tablespoon apple cider vinegar

Directions:

1. Start by preparing the sauce. In a medium bowl, combine sesame oil, minced garlic, grated ginger, erythritol, coconut amino acids, apple cider vinegar and almond butter. Use a whisk to mix everything together vigorously. Cover and refrigerate until cooked through.
2. Now take a large frying pan and place it on heat with a tablespoon of avocado oil. Increase the heat a bit to medium so that the oil gets hot. When the oil is hot, add the ground chicken. Utilize a spatula to break it up while cooking. Let the chicken cook for eight minutes or until lightly browned.
3. When the chicken is cooked, add the onion powder, sea salt and black pepper. Mix everything, and then add the shiitake mushrooms, green onions and jicama. Stir and cook for 5 minutes.
4. Once the mushrooms are soft, after about 5 minutes, pour the sauce over them. Seethe the mixture for 5 minutes then turn off the heat.
5. Take the lettuce with the butter and carefully remove the leaves. Place a sheet on a plate and add a quarter cup of the chicken mixture in the center. Repeat until you have used up the chicken mixture.
6. Serve and enjoy!

Nutritional Facts

Calories 155, Carbs 5g, Fat 5g, Protein 18g

Chicken Pizza Casserole

Prep Time: 13 Min | Cooking Time: 30 Min | Servings: 4

Ingredients

- 1 tablespoon olive oil
- 1 pound boneless chicken thighs
- 2 large zucchini, cubed
- 4 ounces sliced pepperoni, divided
- 12 ounces whole-milk ricotta cheese
- 2 cloves minced garlic
- ¼ cup grated parmesan
- 1 cup shredded mozzarella cheese
- Salt and pepper, to taste

Directions

1. Warm the oven to 350 degrees and grease a 9 x 13-inch glass baking dish.
2. Cook the chicken thighs in a greased pan over medium heat until cooked through.
3. Remove the chicken and place it on a cutting board and chop it with two forks.
4. In a large bowl, combine the grated chicken with the zucchini, ricotta, half the pepperoni, garlic, salt and pepper.
5. Distribute the mixture to the pan and bake for 20 minutes.

6. Sprinkle with mozzarella and Parmesan, and then garnish with remaining peppers.
7. Cook for an additional 5 to 10 minutes until the cheese is melted.

Nutritional Facts:

Calories: 631, Fat 47g, Carbohydrates 7g, Protein 44g, Cholesterol 205 mg

Chicken-Avocado

Salad

Prep Time: 10 Min | Cooking Time: 12 | Servings: 1

Ingredients

- 1 3-ounce boneless chicken thigh
- 1 small celery stalk, diced
- Salt and pepper, to taste
- ½ teaspoon fresh chopped parsley
- 1 tablespoon diced red onion
- 1 cup diced avocado
- Pinch garlic powder
- 1 teaspoon fresh lemon juice
- ⅓ cup sour cream

Directions

1. Grease and preheat a drip pan over medium-high heat.
2. Flavor the chicken with pepper and salt, and then add it to the grill.
3. Cook for 5 to 6 minutes per side until cooked through, then remove it from heat. Allow the chicken to cool slightly then chop it.
4. In a portable bowl, combine the celery, red onion and fresh parsley.
5. Add the diced avocado and the grated chicken.
6. Add sour cream, lemon juice and garlic powder and mix well.

7. Flavor with pepper and salt to taste and serve.

Nutritional Facts:

Calories: 506, Fat 43g, Carbohydrates 6g, Protein 18g, Cholesterol 112 mg

Chili

Prep Time: 11 Min | Cooking Time: 1 hour 45 minutes
| Servings: 3

Ingredients:

- 2 teaspoons erythritol (granulated)
- 3 pounds ground beef
- ⅔ cups celery (diced)
- ½ cup green bell pepper (diced fine)
- ½ cup red bell pepper (diced fine)
- 1 ½ cups yellow bell pepper (diced fine)
- 1 ½ cups tomato juice
- 1 cup tomatoes (diced)
- 1 15-ounce can crushed tomatoes in purée
- 3 tablespoons chili powder
- 3 tablespoons Worcestershire sauce
- 1 teaspoon garlic powder
- ½ teaspoon black pepper
- ½ teaspoon oregano (dried)
- 1 teaspoon cumin
- 1 teaspoon Himalayan sea salt

Directions

1. Take a large saucepan and put it on the heat; turn the heat from medium-high to hot. Include the ground beef to the pot and cook for about 10 minutes or until completely cooked through and dark brown. Stir the meat regularly to avoid lumps. The moment the ground beef is

cooked, drain the excess oil, leaving about 2 tablespoons in the pan.
2. Add the onions, celery, red, green and yellow peppers and diced tomatoes. Stir and cook the peppers for 5 minutes.
3. Then add the tomato juice, crushed tomatoes and Worcestershire sauce. Stir and simmer the liquid for 3 minutes.
4. Add the chili powder, garlic powder, cumin, oregano, sea salt and black pepper to the pot. Blend, lower the heat to medium, cover and cook for 1 hour.
5. After an hour, stir, uncover and cook for another 30 minutes over medium-low heat.
6. Switch off the heat and let the chili stand for about 10 minutes, then pour the ladle into the bowls, top with your favorite seasonings and enjoy!

Nutritional Facts:

Calories 362, Carbs 3g, Fat 11g, Protein 53g

Cinnamon Pork

Prep Time: 11 Min | Cooking Time: 10 Min | Servings: 4

Ingredients:

- A pinch of salt and black pepper
- 2 tablespoons ghee
- 4 pork chops, boneless
- A pinch of nutmeg, ground
- 1 teaspoon cinnamon powder
- 2 tablespoons stevia
- A tablespoon apple cider vinegar

Directions:

1. Heat a pan with the ghee over medium-high heat, add the pork chops and cook for 5 minutes.
2. Flip the chops, season with salt, pepper, stevia, nutmeg and cinnamon, sprinkle with vinegar and cook for another 5 minutes.
3. Divide the ribs between plates and serve for lunch.

Nutritional Facts:

Calories: 261, Fat 4, Carbohydrates 15g, Protein 7g, fiber 7

CHAPTER THREE

Batter-Dipped Fish

Prep Time: 6 Min | Cooking Time: 11 Min | Servings: 3

Ingredients:

- 2 pounds cod (cut into three-inch pieces)
- 4 cups vegetable oil (for frying)
- 16 ounces club soda
- 2 cups almond flour
- ¼ cup ground flaxseed
- ½ teaspoon paprika
- ½ teaspoon baking soda
- ½ teaspoon onion salt
- ½ teaspoon baking powder
- ¼ teaspoon black pepper
- 1 teaspoon Himalayan sea salt

Directions:

1. First, take a deep pan and fill it with the 4 cups of oil. Set the flame to medium to preheat the oil.
2. While the oil is warming, combine the almond flour and ground flax seeds with paprika, onion salt, baking soda, baking powder, sea salt, and

black pepper in a large bowl. Beat everything so that it is well incorporated, then add the club soda. Beat again until the dough is fluffy.

3. Take the pieces of cod and dip them in the batter. Make sure each piece is completely covered, and then gently drop it into the preheated oil. Do not overload the pan, or the fish will not cook evenly. If necessary, fry twice. Fry the fish for 5 minutes. The fish should have a nice golden color, and when it's done, it will start to float in the oil.
4. Take out the fish from the oil with a slotted spoon and transfer it to a paper towel-lined plate to catch excess oil.
5. Serve with your favorite side!

Nutritional Facts:

Calories 559, Carbs 2g, Fat 43g, Protein 37g

Beef and Broccoli

Prep Time: 9 Min | Cooking Time: 25 Min | Servings: 2

Ingredients

- 1 cup broccoli, chopped
- 1 teaspoon coconut oil
- ¼ cup diced yellow onion
- 1 teaspoon fresh grated ginger
- 1 tablespoon soy sauce
- 1 clove minced garlic
- 3 ounces shredded mozzarella cheese
- 12 ounces 80 percent lean ground beef
- 1 large egg
- 2 tablespoons sliced green onion, optional
- Salt and pepper, to taste

Directions

1. In an enormous skillet, heat the coconut oil over high heat.
2. Add the broccoli and onion and sauté for 5 to 7 minutes, until golden brown.
3. Add the soy sauce, ginger, and garlic and sauté for an additional 1 to 2 minutes, until fragrant. Remove from fire.
4. In a separate portable skillet over medium heat, add the ground beef and cook until golden brown; utilize a wooden spoon to break it up. Drain off a little fat.
5. Add the mozzarella and egg and cook until the cheese is melted.

6. Add the broccoli, onion, ginger, and garlic to the meat and mix well.
7. Flavor with pepper and salt to taste; then serve garnished with green onion.

Nutritional Facts:

Calories: 514, Fat 34, Carbohydrates 4g, Protein 45g, Cholesterol 233 mg

Cheesy Brussels Sprout Bake

Prep Time: 14 Min | Cooking Time: 20 Min | Servings: 6

Ingredients

- 3 tbsp. butter
- 5 slices bacon
- 2 small shallots, minced
- Kosher salt
- 2 lb. Brussels sprouts halved
- 1/2 tsp. cayenne pepper
- 1/2 cup shredded Gruyère
- 1/2 cup shredded sharp white cheddar
- 3/4 cup heavy cream

Directions

1. Preheat the oven to 375 °. In an enormous ovenproof skillet over medium heat, cook bacon until crisp, 8 minutes. Drain on a paper towel-lined plate, then chop. Cut the fat off the bacon.
2. Return the pan to medium Warm and melt the butter. Add the shallot and Brussels sprouts and season with salt and cayenne pepper. Cook for about 10 minutes until tender.
3. Take it away from the heat and drizzle with cream, then top with cheese and bacon.

4. Cook until cheese is bubbling, 12 to 15 minutes. (If your cheese is not golden, put it in the oven on the grill and cook for 1 minute.)

Nutritional Facts:

Calories 320, Fat 25g, Carbohydrates 15g, Fiber 6g, Protein 13g

Easy Caprese Chicken

Prep Time: 5 Min | Cooking Time: 35 Min | Servings: 4

Ingredients

- 5 boneless skinless chicken thighs
- 2 tbsp avocado oil
- 6 ounces fresh mozzarella cut into 5 or 6 slices
- 1/4 cup fresh basil chopped
- Salt and pepper
- 1 medium tomato cut into 5 or 6 slices

Directions

1. Preheat the oven to 375F.
2. In an enormous skillet, heat the oil over medium heat until it sparkles. Dredge the chicken thighs with pepper and salt and add a single layer to the pan. Brown the first side until golden, about 2 to 3 minutes, then brown the second side 2 to 3 minutes.
3. Spot the chicken in a single layer in a medium pot or glass baking dish. Top each chicken thigh with a slice of fresh mozzarella, then top each with a slice of tomato.
4. Bake, 25 to 28 minutes, until the cheese is melted and bubbly and the chicken is cooked through. Turn on the grill for 2-3 minutes to brown the top of the cheese.

5. Remove from the oven and sprinkle with fresh basil.

Nutritional Facts

Calories 315, Fat 18.7g, Carbohydrates 1.63g, Fiber 0.4g, Protein 35.7g

Easy Keto Beef Tacos

Prep Time: 18 Min | Cooking Time: 31 Min | Servings: 4

Ingredients

- 1 pound ground beef
- 2 cups shredded Cheddar cheese
- ½ package taco seasoning mix
- ¼ teaspoon ground black pepper
- ½ teaspoon salt
- ½ cup tomatoes, diced
- 1 avocado, diced
- ½ cup shredded Cheddar cheese
- 1 cup shredded lettuce

Directions

1. Warm the oven to 175 ° C. Line two baking sheets with parchment paper or a silicone mat.
2. Roll out the cheddar cheese into four 6-inch circles, 2 inches apart.
3. Bake in the warm oven until cheese is melted and lightly browned, 6 to 8 minutes.
4. Let cool 2 to 3 minutes before lifting with a spatula. Place in the handle of a wooden spoon wrapped in foil balanced over 2 cups/cans. Let the taco shells cool completely, about 10 minutes.

5. Cook the meat until golden brown in a skillet over medium-high heat, frequently stirring to separate meat, about 7 minutes. Season with salt, taco seasoning, and pepper; cook for 1 minute longer.
6. Divide the meat mixture among the taco cheese shells. Top with avocado, lettuce, cheddar cheese, and tomatoes.

Nutritional Facts:

Calories: 676, Carbohydrates: 9.7g, Protein: 40.7g, Fat: 52g, cholesterol 156.9mg

Extra-Crispy Chicken Thighs

Prep Time: 9 Min | Cooking Time: 27 Min | Servings: 2

Ingredients

- 1 tablespoon fresh lemon juice
- 4 boneless chicken thighs, skin on
- Salt and pepper, to taste
- ½ teaspoon garlic powder
- 1 medium zucchini
- 4 tablespoons unsalted butter
- 2 cloves minced garlic
- 1 teaspoon olive oil

Directions

1. Warm the oven to 350 degrees and place a wire rack on a rimmed baking sheet.
2. Brush the chicken thighs with lemon juice, and then sprinkle with garlic powder, salt, and pepper.
3. Spot the chicken thighs on the grill and cook for 20 minutes.
4. In an enormous skillet over medium-high heat, brown the zucchini in olive oil until tender.
5. Add garlic and sauté for another 30 seconds; then season with salt and pepper.
6. Put one tablespoon of butter on each chicken thigh, and then grill until crispy.

7. Serve the chicken with the sautéed zucchini.

Nutritional Facts:

Calories: 867, Fat 66, Carbohydrates 5g, Protein 63g, Cholesterol 426 mg

Keto Chicken Ramen

Prep Time: 10 Min | Cooking Time: 2 hours | Servings: 4

Ingredients

- 12 cups water
- 1 small organic chicken about 3lbs
- 2 organic chicken broth cubes
- 2 tbsp salt
- 4 large eggs
- 2 packs shirataki noodles
- 4 tbsp Gluten-free soy sauce
- 6 green onions chopped

Directions

1. In an enormous saucepan, bring the water to a boil and add the chicken. Lower the heat to medium-low, add the chicken stock cubes and salt. Cover the saucepan and cook for one hour and 15 minutes.
2. Remove the chicken from the pot, leave the broth uncovered and simmer for another 45 minutes over low heat. Once your broth is ready, pass through a colander to remove any impurities.
3. Once your chicken has cooled, remove all the meat from the carcass and place it in a bowl.
4. In a portable saucepan, bring 4 cups of water to a boil and carefully place the four eggs. Cook for

exactly 6 minutes to obtain perfectly fluid egg yolks.
5. For each dish, put half a packet of shirataki noodles, a tablespoon of soy sauce, as much of the chicken as you'd like, a hard-boiled egg cut in half, of course, and a handful of chopped green onions.
6. Serve and enjoy!

Nutritional Facts

Calories: 484, Carbohydrates: 7.6g, Protein: 44g, Fat: 31g, Fiber: 3.2g

Keto Mexican

Shredded Chicken

Prep Time: 12 Min | Cooking Time: 14 Min | Servings: 4

Ingredients

- 1/2 cup diced onion
- 3 Tbsp. butter
- 1 Tbsp. chili powder
- 2 tsp. granulated garlic
- 2 tsp. cumin
- 1 Tbsp. paprika
- 1/3 cup chicken stock or water
- 4 cups cooked chicken (dark & white) shredded or pulled
- 1 tsp. salt
- 8 oz. tomato sauce

Directions

1. In an enormous skillet over medium-high heat, melt the butter and add the chopped onions. Sauté onions until translucent, about 5 to 7 minutes.
2. Add the pieces to the butter and onion and cook for another 30 seconds. Then add the cooked chicken, tomato sauce, and water and mix.

3. Ensure to reduce the heat a bit and simmer for 5 to 10 minutes. Taste and adjust the seasoning as needed.
4. You might probably need more salt if you used water instead of broth. Serve hot over cauliflower rice or in your favorite keto taco shell!

Nutritional Facts

Calories: 126, Carbohydrates: 5g, Protein: 6g, Fat: 9g, Fiber: 2g

CHAPTER FOUR

Almond Bars

Prep Time: 2 hours | Cooking Time: 2 Min | Servings: 4

Ingredients:

- 1 and ¾ cups almond butter
- ¾ cup coconut, unsweetened and shredded
- ¾ cup stevia
- 2 tablespoons coconut oil, melted
- 4 ounces unsweetened dark chocolate, chopped

Directions:

1. In a handy bowl, combine the almond flour with the stevia and coconut and mix well.
2. over medium-low heat, heat a pan and add 1 cup of almond butter and coconut oil, beat well, add this to the almond flour, mix well, transfer to a baking sheet and press well.
3. Heat another pan with the chocolate over medium-high heat, add the rest of the almond

butter, beat well again, pour the latter over the almond mixture and distribute evenly.
4. Refrigerate for 2 hours, cut into 12 bars and serve as an aperitif.

Nutritional Facts:

Calories: 160, Fat 2g, Carbohydrates 8g, Protein 4g, fibers 3

Bacon Brussels Sprouts

Prep Time: 14 Min | Cooking Time: 20 Min | Servings: 6

Ingredients:

- A pinch of salt and black pepper
- 1 pound Brussels sprouts, halved
- 7 bacon slices, chopped
- 2 tablespoons stevia
- 1 yellow onion, chopped
- 2 tablespoons olive oil
- 2 teaspoons sweet paprika
- 1 tablespoon parsley, chopped

Directions:

1. Heat a pan with the oil over medium-high heat, add the onion, stir and sauté for 4 to 5 minutes.
2. Add the bacon, toss and cook for another 3 minutes.
3. Add the sprouts, salt, pepper, stevia, paprika, and parsley, mix, cook for another 10 minutes, divide between plates and serve as a garnish.

Nutritional Facts:

Calories: 261, Fat 4g, Carbohydrates 12g, Protein 9g, fibers 8

Broccoli Snack

Prep Time: 10 minutes | Cooking Time: 20 Min
| Servings: 20

Ingredients:

- 2 cups broccoli florets, steamed for 3 minutes and chopped
- 1 egg
- 1/3 cup cheddar cheese, grated
- 1/3 cup almond flour
- ¼ cup yellow onion, chopped
- A pinch of salt and black pepper
- A drizzle of olive oil
- 2 tablespoons parsley, chopped

Directions:

1. In a handy bowl, mix the broccoli with the egg, cheddar, salt, pepper and parsley, mix, form medium sticks out of this mixture, place them in a pan greased with a little oil, put in the oven at 400 degrees F and bake for 20 minutes.
2. Arrange and serve as a snack on a serving plate.

Nutritional Facts:

Calories: 120, Fat 4g, Carbohydrates 6g, Protein 6g, fibers 2

Buttery Garlic Mushrooms

Prep Time: 13 Min | Cooking Time: 15 Min | Servings: 4

Ingredients

- 1 tablespoon fresh chopped thyme
- ¼ cup unsalted butter, melted
- 1 teaspoon balsamic vinegar
- Salt and pepper, to taste
- Fresh chopped parsley
- 2 cloves minced garlic
- 1½ pounds cremini mushrooms

Directions

1. Warm the oven to 375 degrees and line a rimmed baking sheet with foil.
2. In a medium bowl, combine butter, thyme, vinegar, garlic, salt, and pepper.
3. Toss in the mushrooms until evenly coated.
4. Distribute the mushrooms on the baking sheet and roast for 15 to 20 minutes until tender. Stir halfway through the cooking to help mushrooms cook more evenly.
5. Garnish with parsley to serve.

Nutritional Facts:

Calories: 143, Fat 12g, Carbohydrates 7g, Protein 4g, Cholesterol 31 mg

Cashew Nutty Bars

Prep Time: 10 Min | Cooling Time: 3 hours | Servings: 9

Ingredients

- 1/2 cup Cashews
- 1 cup Almond Flour
- 1/4 cup Keto Maple Syrup
- 1 pinch Salt
- 1/4 cup Butter - melted
- 1/4 cup Shredded Coconut
- 1 tsp. Cinnamon

Directions

1. Combine almond flour and butter in a bowl and mix. Add the grated coconut, maple syrup, cinnamon, and salt. Mix well.
2. Chop a half cup of cashews and add to the mixture.
3. Cover the pan with parchment paper and distribute the dough evenly. Put the bar in the fridge and let it cool for 3 hours.
4. Serve and enjoy!

Nutritional Facts:

Calories: 190, Fat 18g, Carbohydrates 4g, Protein 4g

Cauliflower Mash and Browned Butter

Prep Time: 7 Min | Cooking Time: 20 Min | Servings: 6

Ingredients

- ¾ cups heavy cream
- 1½ pounds cauliflower, chopped
- Salt and pepper, to taste
- 3 ounces unsalted butter
- 1 cup shredded cheddar cheese

Directions

1. Spot the cauliflower in a food processor and mix with the rice-like grains.
2. Pour the cauliflower rice into a large saucepan, then add the cream.
3. Over medium Warm, bring it to a boil and lower the heat, and simmer, about 12-15 minutes until the cauliflower is soft.
4. Flavor with salt and pepper, then add the cheddar cheese. Set it aside.
5. In a portable skillet, melt the butter over medium heat.
6. Cook the butter until it changes to a nice amber color, then sprinkle with mashed cauliflower.

Nutritional Facts:

Calories: 307, Fat 29g, Carbohydrates 4g, Protein 8g, Cholesterol 91 mg

Cheese Chips and Guacamole

Prep Time: 5 minutes | Cooking Time: 12 Min
| Servings: 2

Ingredients

- ¼ teaspoon garlic powder
- ½ cup shredded cheddar cheese
- Pinch cayenne
- ½ small tomato, diced
- 1 medium avocado, chopped
- 1 tablespoon minced white onion
- Salt and pepper, to taste
- 1 tablespoon fresh chopped cilantro
- 1 tablespoon fresh lime juice
- ¼ teaspoon ground cumin

Directions

1. Preheat the oven to 425 degrees and use parchment paper to line a baking sheet.
2. Sprinkle grated cheese in circles on baking sheet, using about 1 tbsp per circle, spacing 1 inch apart.
3. Garnish the cheese with a pinch of garlic powder and cayenne pepper.
4. Bake for 6 to 10 minutes, checking frequently, until the cheese is melted to a boil.
5. Remove from the pan and let cool until crispy.

6. In a bowl, mash the avocado then combine the tomato, onion, lime juice, cilantro and cumin.
7. Season with salt and pepper.
8. Serve the guacamole with the cheddar cheese flakes for dipping.

Nutritional Facts:

Calories: 251, Fat 21g, Carbohydrates 10g, Protein 10g, Cholesterol 30 mg

Cheesy Baked Asparagus

Prep Time: 13 Min | Cooking Time: 30 Min | Servings: 4

Ingredients

- ½ cup heavy cream
- 1½ pounds medium asparagus spears
- Salt and pepper, to taste
- ½ cup grated parmesan cheese
- 1 cup shredded mozzarella cheese

Directions

1. Warm the oven to 400 degrees and grease a 9 x 13-inch glass baking sheet.
2. Remove the ends of the asparagus and place them in the pan. Pour in the cream.
3. Flavor with pepper and salt, then garnish with mozzarella and Parmesan.
4. Bake for approximately 25 minutes until cheese is melted.
5. Place the plate under the grill for 5 minutes to brown the cheese.

Nutritional Facts:

Calories: 249, Fat 20g, Carbohydrates 3g, Protein 13g, Cholesterol 72 mg

Creamy Coleslaw

Prep Time: 11 Min | Cooking Time: 5 Min | Servings: 4

Ingredients

- 1 cup shredded green cabbage
- 4 slices bacon
- 1 cup shredded red cabbage
- ½ cup mayonnaise
- 1 medium carrot, grated
- Pepper, to taste
- 1 tablespoon heavy cream
- ½ teaspoon garlic salt
- 1 teaspoon Dijon mustard

Directions

1. In a portable skillet, cook the bacon over medium-high heat until crisp.
2. Pour the bacon on paper towels to drain, then roughly chop the bacon.
3. Blend the rest of the ingredients in a bowl and mix well.
4. Let cool until ready to serve, then garnish with the chopped bacon.

Nutritional Facts:

Calories: 262, Fat 25g, Carbohydrates 4g, Protein 4g, Cholesterol 26 mg

Curry Stir-Fried Cabbage

Prep Time: 7 Min | Cooking Time: 10 Min | Servings: 4

Ingredients

- ½ small yellow onion, diced
- ¼ cup unsalted butter
- 1½ pounds green cabbage, shredded
- 1 tablespoon red curry paste
- ½ cup fresh chopped cilantro
- 1 tablespoon white wine vinegar
- 2 tablespoons water
- Salt and pepper
- 3 cloves minced garlic

Directions

1. In an enormous skillet, heat the butter over medium-high heat.
2. Add the onions and sauté, 2 to 3 minutes, until golden brown.
3. Add the cabbage and sauté for 5 to 6 minutes, until just tender.
4. Add the vinegar, curry paste, water, garlic, salt, and pepper and sauté for 1 to 2 minutes.
5. Regulate the seasoning to taste and garnish with fresh cilantro to serve.

Nutritional Facts:

Calories: 172, Fat 13g, Carbohydrates 6g, Protein 3g,
Cholesterol 31 mg

Easy Veggie Mix

Prep Time: 11 Min | Cooking Time: 20 Min | Servings: 4

Ingredients:

- 2 carrots, sliced
- 1 pound Brussels sprouts, halved
- 2 tablespoons olive oil
- 1 tablespoon balsamic vinegar
- ½ cup cranberries, dried
- 1 teaspoon rosemary, chopped
- 1 teaspoon thyme, chopped

Directions:

1. Spread the sprouts on a lined baking sheet, add the carrot, rosemary, vinegar, oil, and thyme, and mix. Put it in the oven and bake at 400 degrees for 20 minutes.
2. Divide among plates, sprinkle with blueberries, and serve as a garnish.

Nutritional Facts:

Calories: 199, Fat 2g, Carbohydrates 11g, Protein 7g, fibers 5

Eggplant Fries

Prep Time: 15 Min | Cooking Time: 38 Min | Servings: 4

Ingredients

- 2 cups parmesan cheese - grated
- 4 eggplants
- 1 cup flaxseed
- 8 tbsp. marinara sauce
- 4 tsp oregano (dried)
- 4 tsp basil
- 4 eggs

Directions

1. Preheat the oven to 400 F.
2. Pour the flax seeds into a food processor and mix until powdery. Add the grated Parmesan and mix with the flax flour and herbs.
3. Beat the eggs and add the salt. Cut the eggplant into fries. Dip the fried eggplant in the egg, then the mixture of herbs and flax, and repeat with the egg.
4. Place the fried eggplants on a baking sheet lined with parchment paper and sprinkle with cooking oil. Heat for roughly 15 to 20 minutes or until golden brown.
5. Serve immediately with marinara sauce, and enjoy your meal!

Nutritional Facts:

Calories: 456, Fat 29g, Carbohydrates 8g, Protein 27g

Green Beans and Lemon Cream Sauce

Prep Time: 5 Min | Cooking Time: 4 Min | Servings: 4

Ingredients

- 10 ounces fresh green beans, trimmed
- ¼ cup unsalted butter
- ¼ cup fresh chopped parsley
- Salt and pepper, to taste
- 1 tablespoon fresh lemon zest
- ¼ cup heavy cream

Directions

1. In an enormous skillet, heat the butter over medium-high heat.
2. Add the green beans and sauté for 3-4 minutes, until tender and crisp. Season with salt and pepper to taste.
3. Distribute the beans evenly in the pan and pour the cream over them.
4. Cook over low heat for 1 to 2 minutes, until thickened; then sprinkle with lemon zest and mix.
5. Regulate the seasoning to taste and garnish with parsley to serve.

Nutritional Facts:

Calories: 180, Fat 17g, Carbohydrates 7g, Protein 2g, Cholesterol 51 mg

Italian Cheese Snack

Prep Time: 1 hour | Cooking Time: 10 Min | Servings: 12

Ingredients:

- 1 garlic clove, minced
- Salt and black pepper to the taste
- 2 eggs, whisked
- 8 mozzarella cheese strings, halved
- 1 tablespoon Italian seasoning
- 1 cup parmesan, grated
- ½ cup olive oil

Directions:

1. In a portable bowl, combine the Parmesan with the salt, pepper, Italian seasoning and garlic and mix well.
2. Place the beaten eggs in another bowl.
3. Dip the mozzarella sticks in the egg mixture, then in the cheese mixture, plunge them back into the egg / Parmesan mixture and store in the freezer for 1 hour.
4. Heat a pan with the oil over medium-high heat, add the sticks, fry for 5 minutes on each side, place them in a serving dish and serve.

Nutritional Facts:

Calories: 140, Fat 5g, Carbohydrates 3g, Protein 4g, fiber 1

CHAPTER FIVE

Almond Fudge Brownies

Prep Time: 15 minutes | Cooking Time: 12 Min | Servings: 12 Brownies

Ingredients

- ¾ cup powdered erythritol
- 1 cup almond butter
- 10 tablespoons unsweetened cocoa powder
- ¼ cup stevia-sweetened dark chocolate chips
- 1 teaspoon vanilla extract
- 3 large eggs
- ½ teaspoon baking powder

Directions

1. Warm the oven to 325 degrees and grease a 9x9-inch baking dish with cooking spray.
2. In a food processor, combine the almond butter and erythritol and beat until smooth.
3. Add the cocoa powder, eggs, vanilla, and baking powder to the blender.

4. Blend several times, then blend until smooth.
5. Unfurl the dough in the prepared pan and sprinkle with dark chocolate chips.
6. Cook for 10 to 12 minutes, until solid; then cool completely before slicing to serve.

Nutritional Facts:

Calories: 155, Fat 13g, Carbohydrates 8g, Protein 7g, Cholesterol 47 mg

Avocado Chocolate Mousse

Prep Time: 10 minutes | Cooking Time: 0 Min | Servings: 4

Ingredients

- 2 tablespoons heavy cream
- ½ teaspoon instant coffee powder
- 2 medium avocados
- ¼ cup whipped cream
- 3 tablespoons powdered erythritol
- 2 tablespoons unsweetened cocoa powder
- 1 teaspoon vanilla extract

Directions

1. Dissolve the coffee powder into the heavy cream.
2. Peel the avocados and remove the pits.
3. Pour the avocado pulp into a blender and add the concentration of dissolved coffee, cream, cocoa powder, erythritol, and vanilla extract.
4. Blend until smooth and creamy.
5. Pour into dessert bowls and top with whipped cream to serve.

Nutritional Facts:

Calories: 186, Fat 17g, Carbohydrates 10g, Protein 3g, Cholesterol 21 mg

Banana Almond Muffins

Prep Time: 10 minutes | Cooking Time: 18 Min | Servings: 6

Ingredients

- ⅔ cup powdered erythritol
- 1 cup almond butter
- 3 large eggs
- 1 teaspoon baking powder
- 1½ teaspoons vanilla extract
- ½ teaspoon banana extract
- ¼ cup slivered almonds
- Pinch salt

Directions

1. Warm the oven to 325 degrees and cover half of a muffin pan with parchment paper.
2. In a blender, combine the almond butter and erythritol and beat until smooth.
3. Add the eggs, vanilla, baking powder, banana extract, and salt and beat again until smooth.
4. Divide among the 6 muffin cups.
5. Sprinkle with almonds and bake for 16 to 18 minutes, until solid.

Nutritional Facts:

Calories: 292, Fat 25g, Carbohydrates 8g, Protein 13g, Cholesterol 93 mg

Banana Pudding

Prep Time: 10 minutes | Cooking Time: 5 Min | Servings: 1

Ingredients

- 3 tablespoons powdered erythritol
- ½ cup heavy cream
- 1 large egg yolk
- ½ teaspoon xanthan gum
- 1 teaspoon vanilla extract
- ½ teaspoon banana extract
- ¼ cup sugar-free whipped cream
- Pinch salt

Directions

1. In a double boiler, combine the cream, erythritol, and egg yolk over medium-low heat.
2. Whisk until the erythritol dissolves and the mixture thickens.
3. Include the vanilla and xanthan gum and mix for 1 minute more.
4. Add the banana extract and salt; stir until well combined.
5. Pour into a saucer and cover with plastic, the film touching the pudding.
6. Let it cool for 4 hours, then pour into dessert bowls.
7. Top with whipped cream to serve.

Nutritional Facts:

Calories: 592, Fat 60g, Carbohydrates 7g, Protein 6g, Cholesterol 390 mg

Chocolate Cherry Donuts

Prep Time: 10 minutes | Cooking Time: 15 Min | Servings: 3

Ingredients

- 5 10g bars Dark Choco Perfection
- 2 large Eggs
- 3/4 cup Almond Flour
- 3 tbsp. Coconut Milk (from the carton)
- 1/4 cup Golden Flaxseed Meal
- 3 tbsp. Sweet Perfection
- 1 tsp. Baking Powder
- 2 1/2 tbsp. Coconut Oil
- 1 tsp. Vanilla Extract
- Pinch Salt
- 2 tsp. Berry Extract of Choice

Directions

1. Mix all the wet ingredients into the dough. Cut the chocolate bars into pieces and mix them with the dough. Add the berry extract.
2. Heat your donut maker and lightly grease it. Pour in the batter and cook for 4 to 5 minutes each. Flip each donut and cook for another 2 minutes.
3. Repeat until mixing is complete. Set aside.
4. Serve immediately and enjoy!

Nutritional Facts:

Calories: 106.7, Fat 9.4g, Carbohydrates 6.8g, Protein 3.1g

Chocolate Mousse

Prep Time: 1 hour and 12 minutes | Cooking Time: 0 Min | Servings: 4

Ingredients:

- 1-ounce coconut oil, melted
- 11 ounces dark chocolate, melted
- ½ cup coconut cream
- 1 tablespoon lemon zest, grated
- 1 tablespoon coconut, shredded

Directions:

1. In a portable bowl, combine the melted chocolate with the oil, cream, coconut, and lemon zest, beat well.
2. Divide into bowls and refrigerate for one hour before serving. Enjoy!

Nutritional Facts:

Calories: 173, Fat 12g, Carbohydrates 2g, Protein 3g, fibers 3

Coconut Cookies

Prep Time: 10 minutes | Cooking Time: 20 Min
| Servings: 6

Ingredients:

- ½ cup cocoa chips
- 1 cup almond flour
- ½ cup coconut flakes
- ½ cup almond butter
- 2 eggs
- 1/3 cup stevia
- ¼ cup ghee, melted

Directions:

1. In a portable bowl, combine the flour with the cocoa flakes, coconut flakes, and stevia and mix.
2. Add almond butter, ghee and eggs beat well, place medium cookies on a lined baking sheet, place in the oven and bake at 350 degrees F for 20 minutes.
3. Serve the cookies cold. Enjoy!

Nutritional Facts:

Calories: 200, Fat 12g, Carbohydrates 3g, Protein 5g, fibers 4

Coconut Pies

Prep Time: 10 minutes | Cooking Time: 20 Min | Servings: 4

Ingredients:

- 1 cup stevia
- 4 tablespoons ghee, melted
- ½ cup almond flour
- 1 cup coconut cream
- ¼ cup coconut flakes
- 1 teaspoon vanilla extract
- 2 egg yolks
- ½ cup water
- ¼ cup coconut flour

Directions:

1. Heat a small saucepan with the ghee over medium heat, add half of the stevia, the coconut flakes, and the almond flour, mix, cook for a few minutes, divide into 4 molds and leave to cool.
2. In another saucepan, combine the rest of the stevia with the coconut cream, egg yolks, coconut flour, water, and vanilla extract over medium-low heat, mix for 2 minutes and pour into molds.
3. Let them cool before serving. Enjoy!

Nutritional Facts:

Calories: 231, Fat 12g, Carbohydrates 12g, Protein 9g, fibers 4

Coconut Raspberry Cake

Prep Time: 1 hour and 9 minutes | Cooking Time: 10 Min | Servings: 6

Ingredients:

For the biscuit:

- 1 egg
- 2 cups almond flour
- 1 tablespoon ghee, melted
- For the coconut layer:
- ½ teaspoon baking soda
- 1 cup coconut milk
- 3 cups coconut, shredded
- ¼ cup coconut oil, melted
- 1 teaspoon vanilla extract
- 1/3 cup stevia

For the raspberry layer:

- 1 teaspoon stevia
- 2 tablespoons water
- 1 cup raspberries
- 3 tablespoons chia seeds

Directions:

1. In a portable bowl, mix the almond flour with the eggs, clarified butter, and baking soda, mix

well, press the bottom of the mold into a spring, put it in the oven at 350 degrees for 15 minutes, and set it aside to cool down.
2. Meanwhile, in a frying pan, mix the raspberries with 1 teaspoon of stevia, the chia seeds, and the water, mix, cook for 5 minutes, remove from the heat, allow it to cool, and spread over the layer of biscuit.
3. In another saucepan, combine the coconut milk with the coconut oil, 1/3 cup of stevia, and the vanilla extract, mix for 1 to 2 minutes, remove from the heat, cool, and spread over the coconut milk.
4. Put the cake in the refrigerator and chill for 1 hour, slice it and serve. Enjoy!

Nutritional Facts:

Calories: 241, Fat 12g, Carbohydrates 5g, Protein 5g, fibers 4

Creamy Cookie Dough Mousse

Prep Time: 10 minutes | Cooking Time: 3 Min | Servings: 2

Ingredients

- 4 ounces cream cheese, softened
- 2 tablespoons unsalted butter
- ¼ cup stevia-sweetened dark chocolate chips
- ¼ cup powdered erythritol
- 1½ teaspoons vanilla extract
- 1 teaspoon sugar-free maple syrup

Directions

1. In a portable saucepan, melt the butter over low heat until golden brown.
2. In a medium bowl, combine cream cheese, erythritol, maple syrup, and vanilla extract with a hand mixer until smooth and blended.
3. Beat the golden butter until the mixture is smooth and well combined.
4. Fold in the chocolate chips, then pour into two dessert bowls and refrigerate until ready to serve.

Nutritional Facts:

Calories: 378, Fat 37g, Carbohydrates 16g, Protein 5g, Cholesterol 93 mg

Delicious Brownies

Prep Time: 10 Min | Cooking Time: 25 Min | Servings: 4

Ingredients:

- 4 tablespoons ghee, melted
- ¼ cup cocoa powder
- 5 ounces chocolate, melted
- 3 eggs
- ¼ cup mascarpone cheese
- ½ cup swerve

Directions:

1. In a portable bowl, mix the melted chocolate with the clarified butter, eggs, vinegar, cheese, and cocoa, beat well, pour into a saucepan, put in the oven, and bake at 375 degrees for 25 minutes.
2. Cut into medium brownies and serve. Enjoy!

Nutritional Facts:

Calories: 120, Fat 8g, Carbohydrates 3g, Protein 3g, fibers 4

Easy Cinnamon Mug Cake

Prep Time: 5 minutes | Cooking Time: 10 Min | Servings: 1

Ingredients

- ¾ teaspoon ground cinnamon, divided
- 2 tablespoons powdered erythritol, divided
- ¼ cup almond flour
- Pinch salt
- Sugar-free maple syrup
- ¼ teaspoon ground nutmeg
- 1 large egg
- ½ teaspoon vanilla extract
- 1 tablespoon unsalted butter, melted

Directions

1. In a small bowl, mix ½ tablespoon of erythritol with ¼ teaspoon of cinnamon and set it aside.
2. Turn on the oven and preheat to 350 degrees and grease a 4-ounce pan with cooking spray.
3. In a small bowl, combine the almond flour with the remaining erythritol, remaining cinnamon, nutmeg, and salt until combined.
4. Add egg, butter, and vanilla extract until smooth.

5. Pour the mixture into the greased plate and sprinkle with the erythritol and cinnamon mixture.
6. Bake for 12 minutes (or microwave over high heat for 1 minute) until solid
7. Drizzle with unsweetened maple syrup and serve in the baking dish

Nutritional Facts:

Calories: 349, Fat 31g, Carbohydrates 11g, Protein 13g, Cholesterol 217 mg

CONCLUSION

I hope so much that you enjoyed preparing and cooking these fantastic dishes, designed for you.

Remembering that the ketogenic diet is always recommended for short periods, it is always better to talk to a nutritionist before starting it and continue for a long time, always keeping blood values under control.

Thank you for reading, and have fun with the recipes.

CPSIA information can be obtained
at www.ICGtesting.com
Printed in the USA
BVHW041010150321
602551BV00006B/353